Your smart device plus this book equals a first aid course in your hands.

First Aid for New Parents helps eliminate the guesswork when attempting to decipher an infant's cries, coughs, breathing and appearance when an infant is ill. As infants grow and become more mobile, the potential for an accidental injury rises and parents need to prepare themselves to treat life threatening injuries and illnesses while they wait on EMS to arrive.

I read and researched textbooks from the major first responder medical training schools and consolidated thousands of pages of text into intuitive, easy-to-use flow diagrams that graphically illustrate first aid treatment and care.

You will learn how to:

- Decipher infants coughs and unusual breathing sounds. Point your cell phone camera towards the QR Codes found in the book to listen to examples of coughs and unusual breathing. You can then follow a flow diagram that will walk you step-by-step in understanding if your infant requires immediate medical attention.
- Treat common infant illnesses and injuries.
- Understand when an illness or injury requires immediate medical attention

First Aid for New Parents goes another step further by enabling you to view over 30 presentations and demonstrations on your smart device. Each page of this book is explained, step-by-step in using concise, to the point video presentations. Video demonstrations throughout the book will deepen your knowledge by illustrating the application of first aid concepts. Enable the QR Code reader on your smart device and point your smart device's camera at the QR Code found on pages throughout this book. You will be directed to engaging video demonstrations and classroom lectures.

The book is excellent for parents, grandparents, daycare professionals, church nursery volunteers, nannies and babysitters.

My life mission is to teach people with no medical background how they can save lives in the first critical minutes of a medical emergency and care for the ill and injured while waiting for EMS to arrive.

Jeffrey S. Imel
jeff@udtwfa.com
Fishers, Indiana
January 2021

Infant Primary Assessment

(1)

Primary Assessment

START → Scene Size-Up / Scene Safety / General Impression → Do you see life threatening bleeding?

- Yes → **(20)** Bleeding Control
- No →

Awake — Is the infant responsive or crying?

- Yes → **Airway.** Open the infant's airway by slightly tilting the infant's head back.
- No → Tap on the bottom of the infant's foot and say the infant's name. Is the infant responsive?
  - Yes → **Airway.** Open the infant's airway by slightly tilting the infant's head back.
  - No → **Airway.** Open the infant's airway by slightly tilting the infant's head back.

If you witness an infant collapse and go unresponsive - immediately call 911 and begin CPR

Breathing — Place your ear close to the infant's mouth and listen for breathing. Look at the infant's torso and look for rise and fall. Note if breathing sounds abnormal.

Breathing — Place your ear close to the infant's mouth and listen for breathing. Look at the infant's torso and look for rise and fall. Note if breathing sounds abnormal. Is the infant breathing?

- No → **(6)** CPR
- Yes →

Is the infant presenting with abnormal breathing or breathing difficulty?

- Yes → **(8)** Abnormal Breathing
- No →

Circulation — Check the infant for bleeding. Check under the infant using your gloved hand, looking for blood on your glove. Do you see any bleeding?

- Yes → **(20)** Bleeding Control
- No → **(2)** Infant Secondary Assessment

First Aid for New Parents

Copyright © 2021 by UDTWFA, LLC

ISBN: 978-1-7335440-8-5

The procedures and protocols in this book are based on the most current recommendations of responsible medical sources. The author and the publisher, however, make no guarantee as to, and assume no responsibility for, the correctness, sufficiency or completeness of such information or recommendations. Furthermore, the author and the publisher do not assume and hereby disclaim any liability for loss, damage, injury or disruption caused by errors, or omissions, whether such omissions result from negligence, accident or any other cause. Other or additional safety measures may be required under particular circumstances. Use of this publication does not create a physician-patient relationship. You are solely responsible for your decision to obtain treatment from a medical professional.

This publication is designed for educational purposes only and not for the purpose of rendering medical advice. The information presented through this publication is not intended to replace the counsel of a physician. It is not intended as a statement of the standards of care required in any particular situation, because circumstances and the patient's physical condition can vary widely from one emergency to another. Nor is it intended that this book shall in any way advise people responding to emergency situations concerning legal authority to perform the activities or procedures discussed.

Table of Contents

Infant Secondary Assessment

LIFE THREAT

CALL 911 FOR AN INFANT WITH A SERIOUS INJURY FOUND IN THE SECONDARY ASSESSMENT OR IF YOU ARE CONCERNED ABOUT THE INFANT.

Cervical Spine
Hold the infant's head to maintain in-line stabilization. Gently palpate the cervical vertebrae and note any cervical spine pain, tenderness or deformity. Check the soft tissues for bruising, pain and tenderness.

Buttocks
Look for any soft-tissue injury such as bruising, bleeding or lacerations.

Limbs
Inspect all the limbs and joints. Palpate for bony and soft-tissue tenderness and check joint movements, stability and muscular power. Note any bruising or lacerations and evidence of muscle, nerve or tendon damage. Look for any deformities, penetrating injuries or open fractures.

Call 911 for any injury found during the Primary or Secondary Assessments.

Neck
Check - Trachea is in-line or is it pushing off to one side? Check - Any blood vessels bulging?

Chest
Inspect the chest. Look for any bruising, lacerations, penetrating injury or tenderness.

Abdomen
Inspect the abdomen looking for distension, bruising, laceration or penetrating injury.

Pelvis
Gently palpate for any tenderness.

Spine
Log roll the infant. Maintain in-line stabilisation throughout. Inspect the entire length of the back noting any bruising or lacerations. Palpate the spine for any tenderness or fractured vertebrae.

1 **Infant Primary Assessment**

Head
Inspect the scalp. Look for any bleeding or lacerations.

Assess the fontanelles in infant. A bulging fontanelle may be a sign of raised intracranial pressure.

Eyes
Examine the eyes for any foreign body, subconjunctival hemorrhage, hyphema, irregular iris, penetrating injury or contact lenses.

Ears
Examine the ears for any bruising behind the ear, bleeding as well as any cerebrospinal fluid (CSF) leak.

Nose
Examine the nose for any deformities, bleeding and CSF leak. Do not plug nose to stop leak.

Mouth
Examine the mouth for cuts to the lips, gums, tongue or palate. Inspect teeth, noting if any are loose, missing or fractured.

SAMPLE History

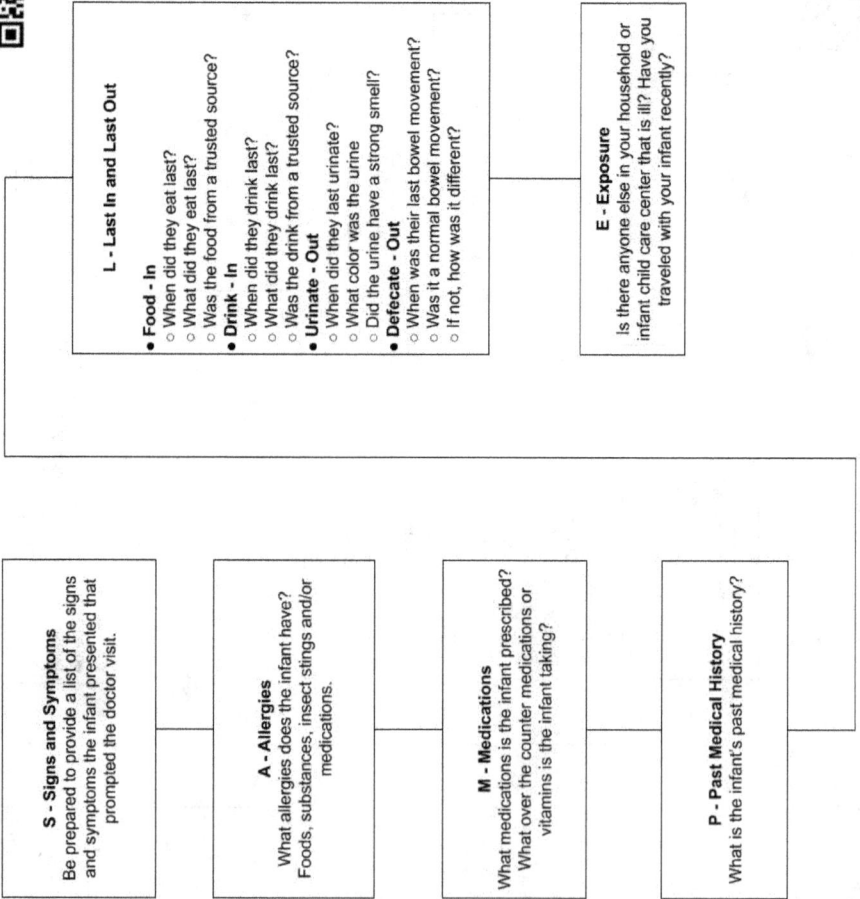

L - Last In and Last Out

- **Food - In**
  - When did they eat last?
  - What did they eat last?
  - Was the food from a trusted source?
- **Drink - In**
  - When did they drink last?
  - What did they drink last?
  - Was the drink from a trusted source?
- **Urinate - Out**
  - When did they last urinate?
  - What color was the urine
  - Did the urine have a strong smell?
- **Defecate - Out**
  - When was their last bowel movement?
  - Was it a normal bowel movement?
  - If not, how was it different?

E - Exposure

Is there anyone else in your household or infant child care center that is ill? Have you traveled with your infant recently?

S - Signs and Symptoms

Be prepared to provide a list of the signs and symptoms the infant presented that prompted the doctor visit.

A - Allergies

What allergies does the infant have? Foods, substances, insect stings and/or medications.

M - Medications

What medications is the infant prescribed? What over the counter medications or vitamins is the infant taking?

P - Past Medical History

What is the infant's past medical history?

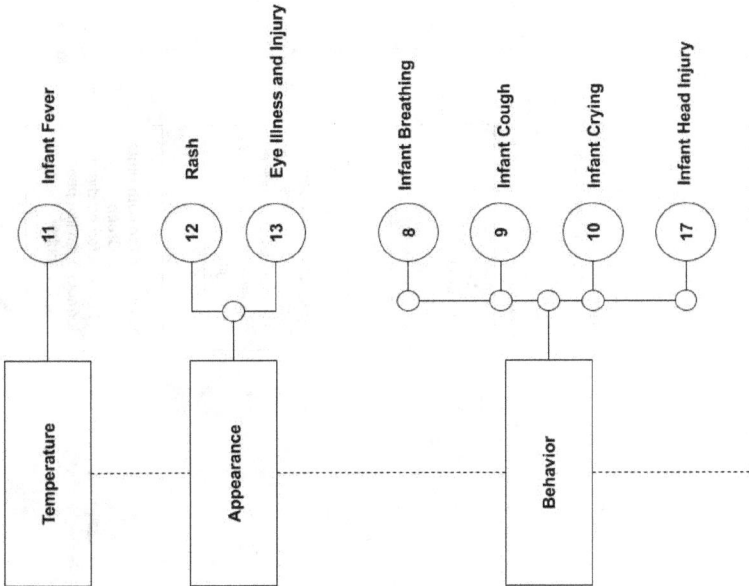

Temperature

(11) Infant Fever

Appearance

(12) Rash

(13) Eye Illness and Injury

Behavior

(8) Infant Breathing

(9) Infant Cough

(10) Infant Crying

(17) Infant Head Injury

Input/Output

Contact the doctor for any one of the following

Changes in Appetite
If the infant refuses several feedings in a row or eats poorly.

Diarrhea
The infant's stools are especially loose or watery.

Vomiting
The infant vomits forcefully after feedings or if the infant hasn't been able to keep liquids down for eight hours.

Dehydration
Infant cries with fewer tears, has significantly fewer wet diapers, has a dry mouth or soft spot appears sunken.

Constipation
The infant has fewer bowel movements than usual for a few days and appears to be struggling or uncomfortable.

Bowel Movements
See Infant Poop Color diagrams on page 5.

Poison
If you believe the infant has ingested poison.

CALL 911 IMMEDIATELY FOR ANY OF THE FOLLOWING

- Bleeding that can't be stopped
- Poisoning
- Seizures
- Increasing difficulty breathing
- Any change in consciousness, confusion, a bad headache or vomiting several times after a head injury
- Unconsciousness, acting strangely or becoming more withdrawn and less alert
- Large or deep cuts or burns or smoke inhalation
- Skin or lips that look blue, purple or gray
- Increasing or severe persistent pain
- Major mouth or facial injuries
- Near drowning
- If you have any concerns and believe you should call 911

Infant Poop Color

Black or dark green
After birth, a baby's first bowel movements are black and tarry.

Yellow-green
Normal color as the baby begins digesting breast milk.

Yellow
(Light Mustard Color)
Normal color for breastfed newborns. Loose bowel movements that look like light mustard.

Yellow or Tan with hints of Green
Formula fed newborn formula. Frim like peanut butter.

See Doctor Immediately for Poop That Is
- Still black several days after birth
- Red or bloody
- White
- Suddenly more frequent and unusually watery
- Less frequent than what is normal for the infant
- Consistently hard, dry and difficult to pass

If you're concerned about the color or consistency of your baby's bowel movements, contact the doctor immediately.

Infant CPR

⑥

Primary Survey ①

Call 911
Have bystander call 911. If alone, call 911 on cell phone and place on speaker mode.

Chest Compressions
Place two fingers in the center of the baby's chest and push down approximatley 1.5 inches. Release the pressure allowing the chest to come back up.

Repeat this 30 times at a rate of 100 to 120 compressions per minute.

Rescue Breaths
Open the airway and give two puffs.

Continue CPR
Keep alternating 30 compressions with two puffs (30:2) until EMS arrives and takes over or the infant starts showing signs of life and starts to breathe normally.

If the infant shows signs of becoming responsive, such as, coughing, opening their eyes, making a noise, or starts to breathe normally, put them in the recovery position.

Monitor their level of response and prepare to give CPR again if necessary. Infant requires immediate medical care.

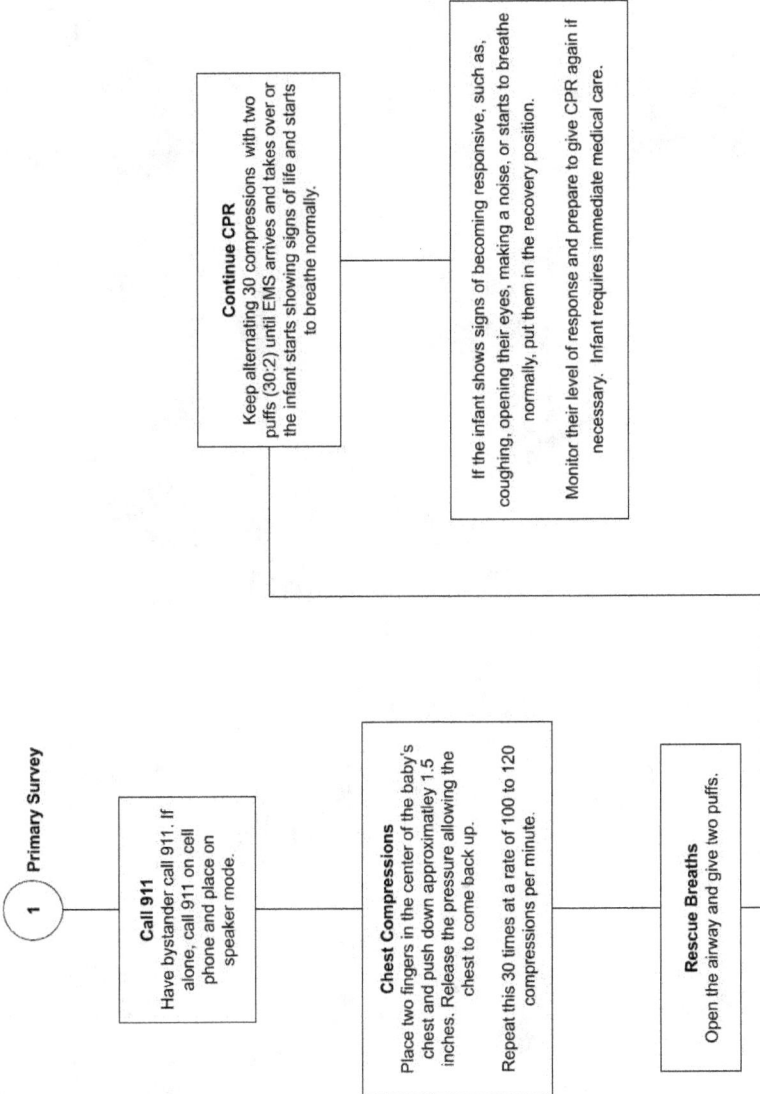

Choking

LIFE THREAT
HAVE BYSTANDER CALL 911 WHILE YOU TREAT FOR CHOKING

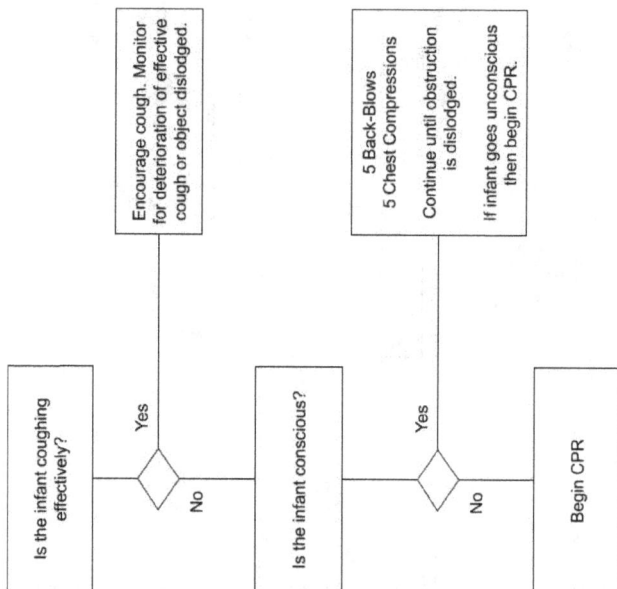

Is the infant coughing effectively?

Yes → Encourage cough. Monitor for deterioration of effective cough or object dislodged.

No

Is the infant conscious?

Yes → 5 Back-Blows
5 Chest Compressions

Continue until obstruction is dislodged.

If infant goes unconscious then begin CPR.

No

Begin CPR

Infant breathing

CALL 911 IMMEDIATELY FOR ANY INFANT THAT IS

- Wheezing rapidly
- Grunting
- Unable to catch their breath
- Turning blue
- Rapidly retracting and expanding their stomach

Seek immediate medical attention if :
- Difficulty in breathing
- High fever
- Blue color to the skin, lips or the nail beds.

Treatment
Provide infant with fluids, rest and cool-mist humidifier. Monitor breathing rate. Contact doctor if you are concerned.

Seek immediate medical attention.

Treatment
Suction nostrils.

Newborns are nose breathers. Possible obstruction in nostrils.

Respiratory Syncytial Virus (RSV)
Usually seen - fall and winter
Possible slight fever.

Signs and Symptoms
One or More of the Following:
- Flaring nostrils
- Retractions - chest and neck visibly moving in and out
- Grunting
- Cyanosis - skin turning blue

Seek immediate medical attention.

(7) **Choking**

Gasping or Coughing
Especially when eating.

Whistling Noise

Wheezing

Labored Breathing

Fast Breathing
Greater than 50 breaths per minute. Labored breathing.

Infant Cough ⑨

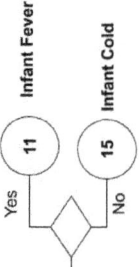

LIFE THREAT
INFANT LESS THAN FOUR MONTHS OLD WITH A COUGH REQUIRES IMMEDIATE MEDICAL ATTENTION

CALL 911 IMMEDIATELY FOR ANY INFANT THAT IS

- Wheezing rapidly
- Grunting
- Unable to catch their breath
- Turning blue
- Rapidly retracting and expanding their stomach

---

⑦ **Choking**

Gasping or Coughing Especially when eating

Does the infant have a temperature 100.4 degrees of higher?

Yes — ⑪ **Infant Fever**

No — ⑮ **Infant Cold**

Dry Hack

Seek immediate medical attention

Whooping Cough
Loud, rapid "woop" with frequent coughing spasms

Seek immediate medical attention

Pneumonia
Cough - Wet and Phlegmy
Coughing up mucus that is green and yellow tinged.

Wet Cough
May present with phlegm or mucus - sometimes with blood.

Seek immediate medical attention

Grunting

If cough does not clear up in a few days or gets worse, seek immediate medical attention

Treatment
Allow your child to breathe moist air
- Damp air from shower
- Cool evening air
- Cool mist humidifier

Croup
Barking noise on inhale.
Worsens at night.

Barking Cough

Seek immediate medical attention

Abnormal, high-pitched sound when breathing in. Possibly Drooling, anxious, restless behavior

Stridor

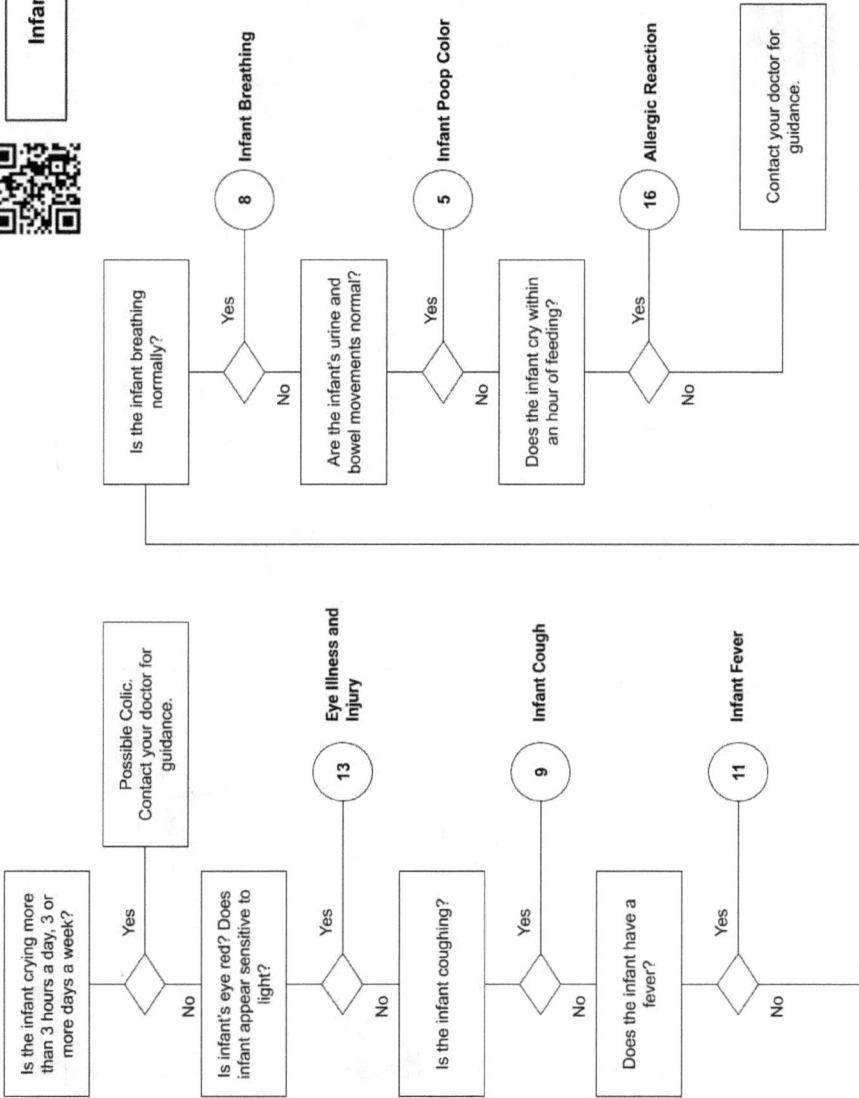

Infant Breathing (8)

Is the infant breathing normally?
- Yes → Infant Breathing (8)
- No → Are the infant's urine and bowel movements normal?

Infant Poop Color (5)

Are the infant's urine and bowel movements normal?
- Yes → Infant Poop Color (5)
- No → Does the infant cry within an hour of feeding?

Allergic Reaction (16)

Does the infant cry within an hour of feeding?
- Yes → Allergic Reaction (16)
- No → Contact your doctor for guidance.

Is the infant crying more than 3 hours a day, 3 or more days a week?
- Yes → Possible Colic. Contact your doctor for guidance.
- No → Is infant's eye red? Does infant appear sensitive to light?

Eye Illness and Injury (13)

Is infant's eye red? Does infant appear sensitive to light?
- Yes → Eye Illness and Injury (13)
- No → Is the infant coughing?

Infant Cough (9)

Is the infant coughing?
- Yes → Infant Cough (9)
- No → Does the infant have a fever?

Infant Fever (11)

Does the infant have a fever?
- Yes → Infant Fever (11)
- No →

Infant Fever

Contact your doctor or call 911 if you have any concerns about your infant.

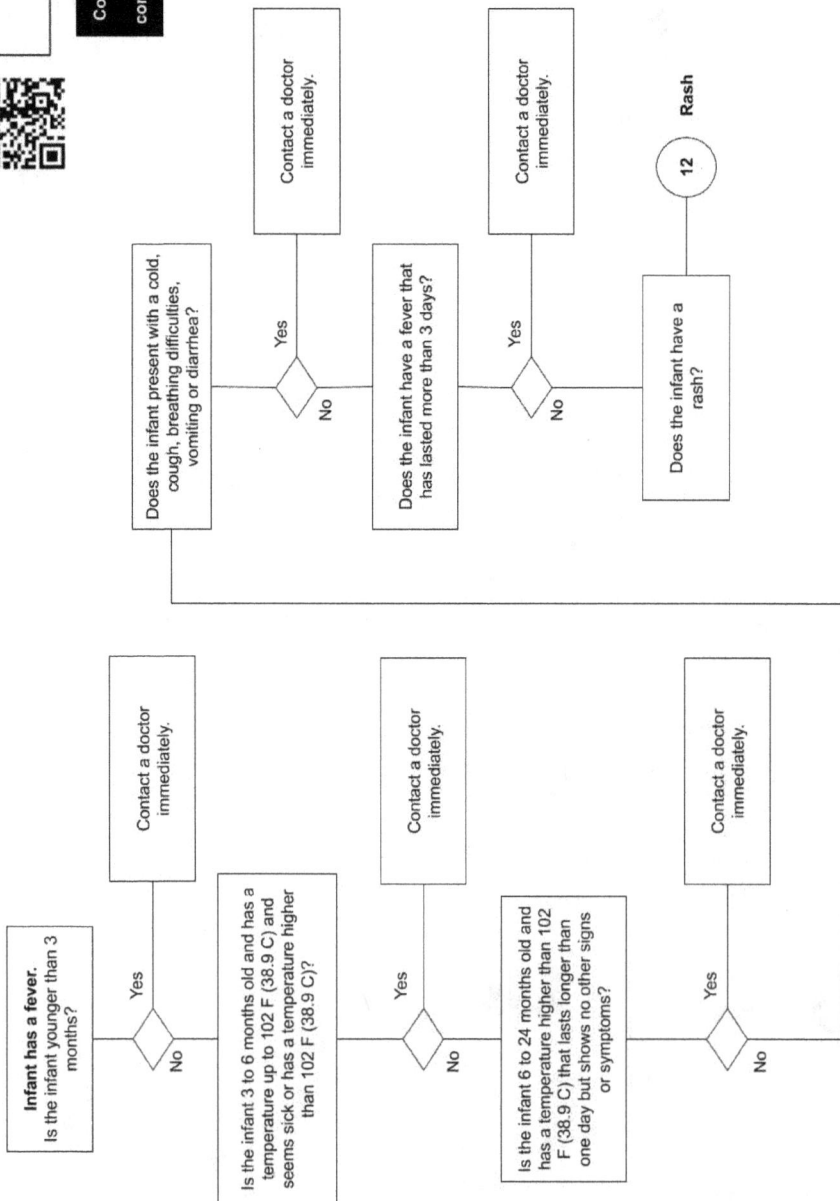

Infant has a fever.
Is the infant younger than 3 months?

Yes → Contact a doctor immediately.

No →

Is the infant 3 to 6 months old and has a temperature up to 102 F (38.9 C) and seems sick or has a temperature higher than 102 F (38.9 C)?

Yes → Contact a doctor immediately.

No →

Is the infant 6 to 24 months old and has a temperature higher than 102 F (38.9 C) that lasts longer than one day but shows no other signs or symptoms?

Yes → Contact a doctor immediately.

No →

Does the infant present with a cold, cough, breathing difficulties, vomiting or diarrhea?

Yes → Contact a doctor immediately.

No →

Does the infant have a fever that has lasted more than 3 days?

Yes → Contact a doctor immediately.

No →

Does the infant have a rash?

12 Rash

Infant Rash

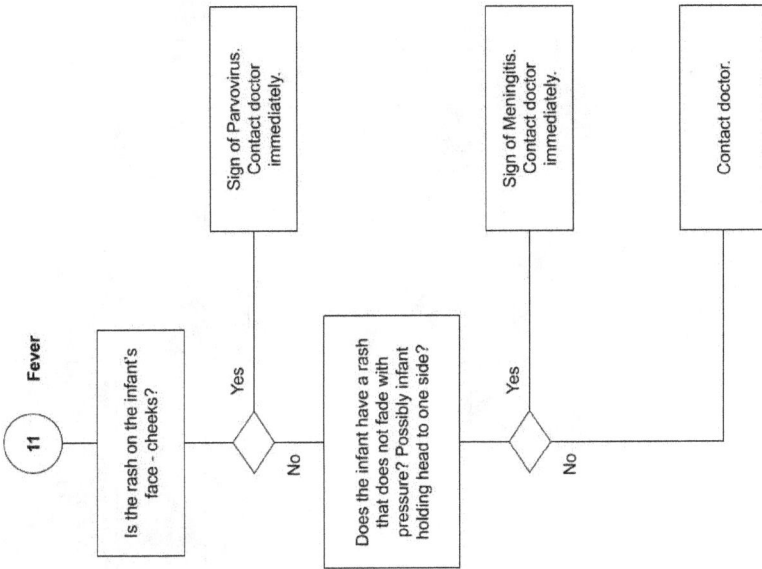

Fever

11

Is the rash on the infant's face - cheeks?

— Yes → Sign of Parvovirus. Contact doctor immediately.

— No →

Does the infant have a rash that does not fade with pressure? Possibly infant holding head to one side?

— Yes → Sign of Meningitis. Contact doctor immediately.

— No → Contact doctor.

Eye Illness and Injury

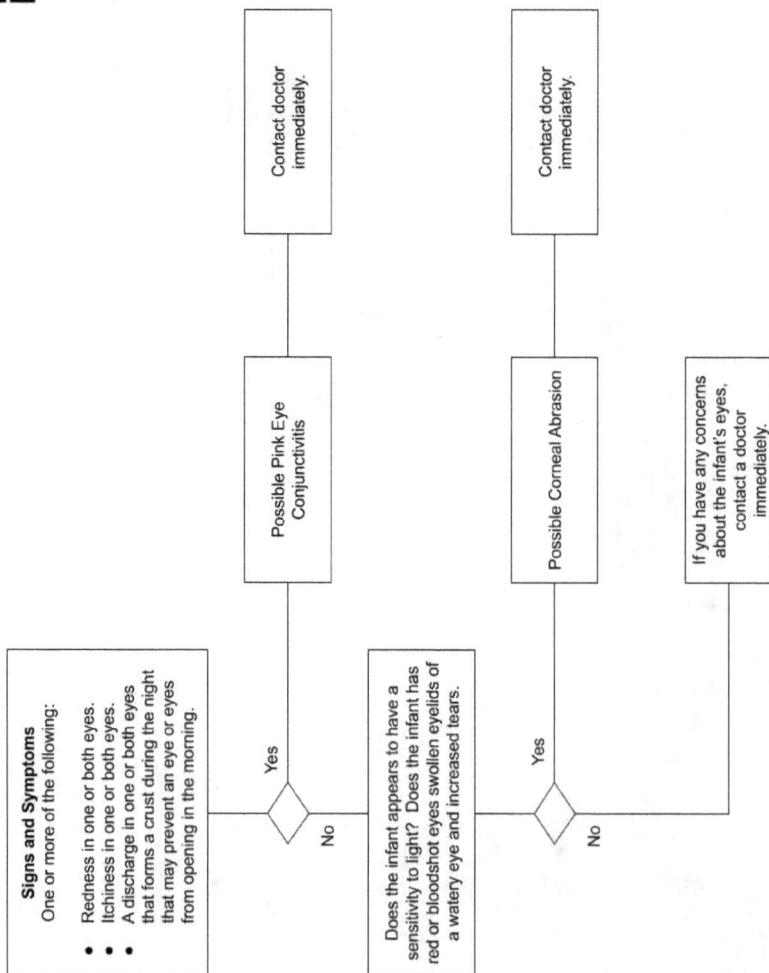

Signs and Symptoms
One or more of the following:

- Redness in one or both eyes.
- Itchiness in one or both eyes.
- A discharge in one or both eyes that forms a crust during the night that may prevent an eye or eyes from opening in the morning.

Yes → Possible Pink Eye Conjunctivitis → Contact doctor immediately.

No →

Does the infant appears to have a sensitivity to light? Does the infant has red or bloodshot eyes swollen eyelids of a watery eye and increased tears.

Yes → Possible Corneal Abrasion → Contact doctor immediately.

No → If you have any concerns about the infant's eyes, contact a doctor immediately.

Ear Infection

Signs and Symptoms
One or more of the following
- Ear pain, especially when lying down
- Tugging or pulling at an ear
- Trouble sleeping
- Crying more than usual
- Fussiness
- Trouble hearing or responding to sounds
- Loss of balance
- Fever of 100 F (38 C) or higher
- Drainage of fluid from the ear
- Headache
- Loss of appetite

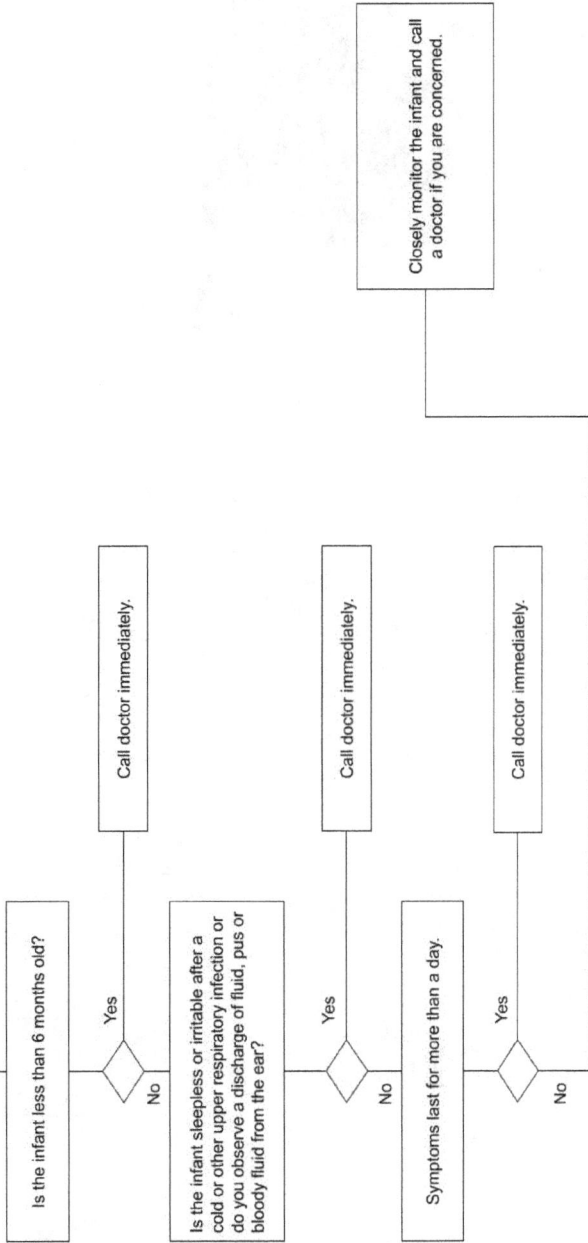

Is the infant less than 6 months old?

Yes → Call doctor immediately.

No ↓

Is the infant sleepless or irritable after a cold or other upper respiratory infection or do you observe a discharge of fluid, pus or bloody fluid from the ear?

Yes → Call doctor immediately.

No ↓

Symptoms last for more than a day.

Yes → Call doctor immediately.

No → Closely monitor the infant and call a doctor if you are concerned.

Infant Cold

A congested or runny nose. Nasal discharge that may be clear at first but might thicken and turn yellow or green

Is infant younger than 3 months of age?

No → Yes → Call doctor.

Does the infant have one or more of the following:
- Not wetting as many diapers as usual
- Has a temperature higher than 100.4 F (38 C)
- Appears to have ear pain or is unusually irritable
- Red eyes or develops yellow or greenish eye discharge
- Trouble breathing
- Persistent cough
- Thick, green nasal discharge for several days
- Unusual or alarming cry
- Has other signs or symptoms that worry you.

Yes → Call doctor.

No → Closely monitor the infant and contact doctor immediately if you are concerned.

LIFE THREAT
INFANT REQUIRES IMMEDIATE MEDICAL ATTENTION FOR ANY ONE OF THE FOLLOWING
- Refuses to nurse or accept fluids
- Coughs hard enough to cause vomiting or changes in skin color
- Coughs up blood-tinged sputum
- Has difficulty breathing or is bluish around the lips

Allergic Reaction

**LIFE THREAT
SEVERE ALLERGIC REACTION
ANAPHYLAXIS**

Signs and symptoms may include:

- Constriction of airways
- Swelling of the throat that makes it difficult to breathe
- A severe drop in blood pressure (shock)
- Rapid pulse
- Loss of consciousness

Do you have an EpiPen?

Yes → Administer EpiPen. Call 911.

No → Call 911.

Mild Allergic Reaction

- Hives
- Wheezing
- Itching or tingling feeling around the lips or mouth
- Swelling of the lips, tongue or throat
- Coughing or shortness of breath
- Vomiting

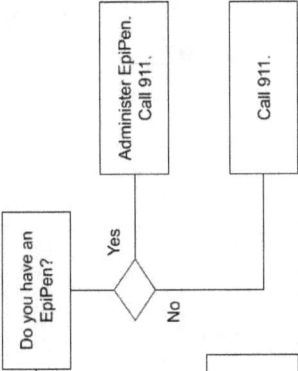

Has the infant has been stung by a bee?

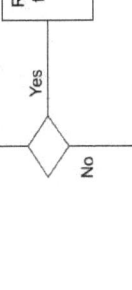

Yes → Remove the stinger by flicking the stinger off with the edge of a credit card. → Monitor the infant closely. Stand by with infant's EpiPen if prescribed. Be prepared to call 911 if allergic reaction turns severe.

No

Has the infant ate or drank anything within a few minutes to a few hours of the above signs and symptoms appearing?

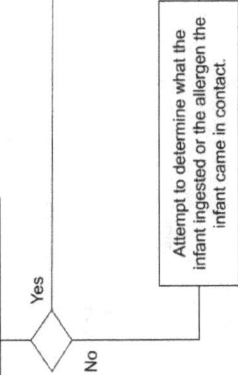

Yes → Consider Milk Allergy. Other signs and symptoms Include:

- Loose stools or diarrhea, which may contain blood
- Abdominal cramps
- Runny nose
- Watery eyes
- Colic

→ Monitor the infant closely. Contact doctor to discuss possible milk allergy.

No → Attempt to determine what the infant ingested or the allergen the infant came in contact. → Monitor the infant closely. Contact doctor to discuss possible allergy.

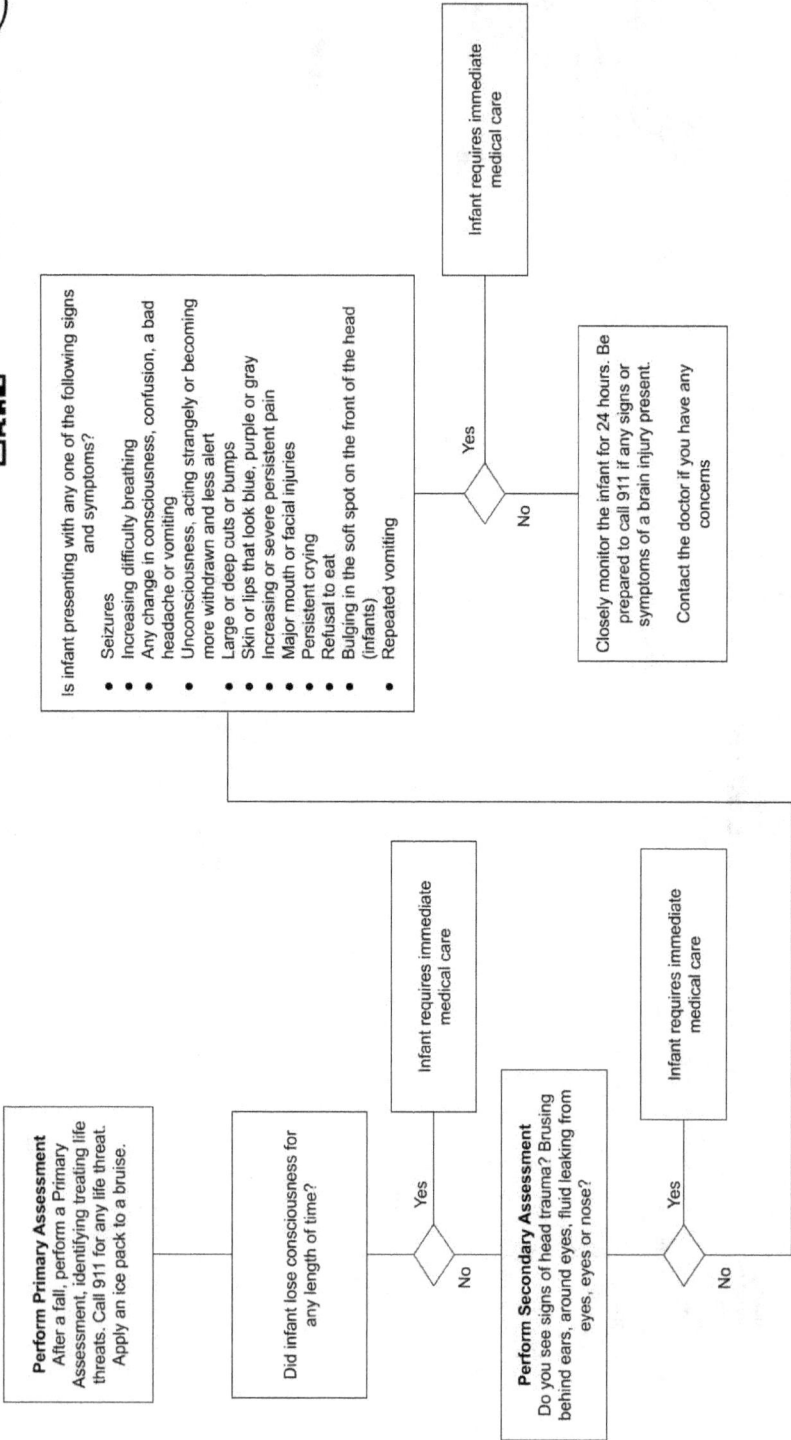

Perform Primary Assessment
After a fall, perform a Primary Assessment, identifying treating life threats. Call 911 for any life threat. Apply an ice pack to a bruise.

Did infant lose consciousness for any length of time?

Yes → Infant requires immediate medical care

No

Perform Secondary Assessment
Do you see signs of head trauma? Brusing behind ears, around eyes, fluid leaking from eyes, eyes or nose?

Yes → Infant requires immediate medical care

No

Is infant presenting with any one of the following signs and symptoms?

- Seizures
- Increasing difficulty breathing
- Any change in consciousness, confusion, a bad headache or vomiting
- Unconsciousness, acting strangely or becoming more withdrawn and less alert
- Large or deep cuts or bumps
- Skin or lips that look blue, purple or gray
- Increasing or severe persistent pain
- Major mouth or facial injuries
- Persistent crying
- Refusal to eat
- Bulging in the soft spot on the front of the head (infants)
- Repeated vomiting

Yes → Infant requires immediate medical care

No

Closely monitor the infant for 24 hours. Be prepared to call 911 if any signs or symptoms of a brain injury present.

Contact the doctor if you have any concerns

Extremity Injury

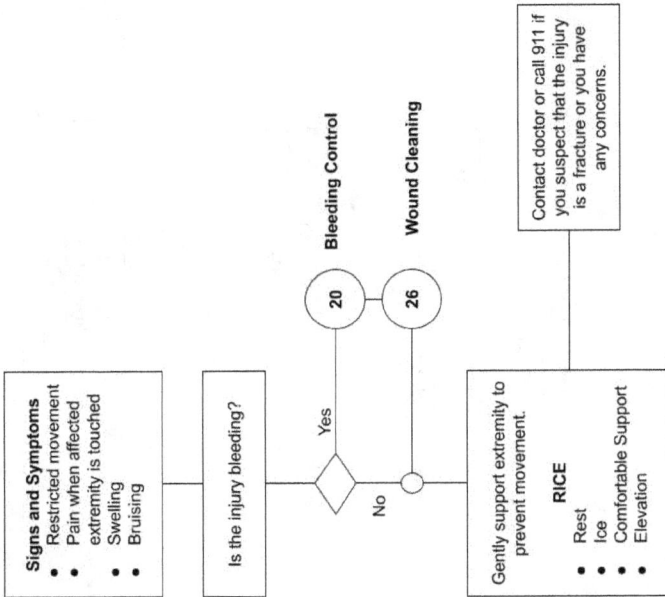

Signs and Symptoms
- Restricted movement
- Pain when affected extremity is touched
- Swelling
- Bruising

Is the injury bleeding?

Yes

20 Bleeding Control

26 Wound Cleaning

No

Gently support extremity to prevent movement.

RICE
- Rest
- Ice
- Comfortable Support
- Elevation

Contact doctor or call 911 if you suspect that the injury is a fracture or you have any concerns.

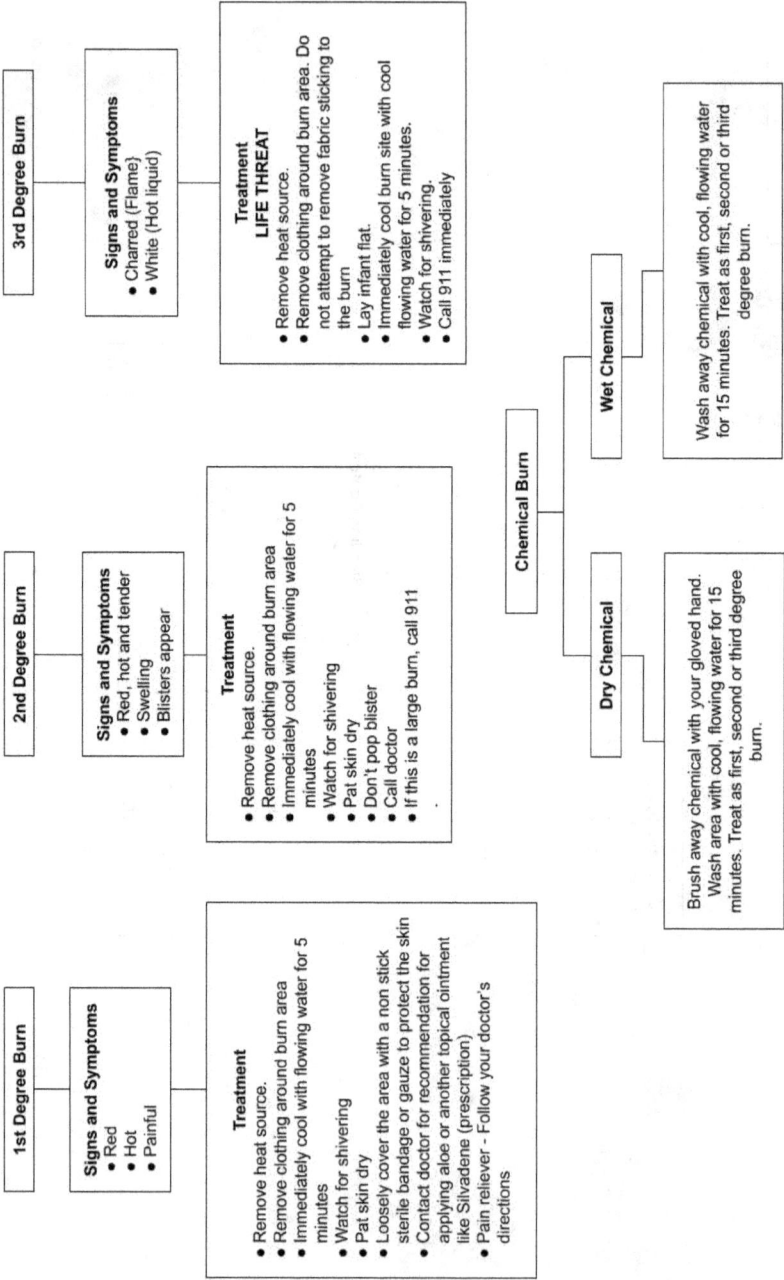

Burns

1st Degree Burn

Signs and Symptoms
- Red
- Hot
- Painful

Treatment
- Remove heat source.
- Remove clothing around burn area
- Immediately cool with flowing water for 5 minutes
- Watch for shivering
- Pat skin dry
- Loosely cover the area with a non stick sterile bandage or gauze to protect the skin
- Contact doctor for recommendation for applying aloe or another topical ointment like Silvadene (prescription)
- Pain reliever - Follow your doctor's directions

2nd Degree Burn

Signs and Symptoms
- Red, hot and tender
- Swelling
- Blisters appear

Treatment
- Remove heat source.
- Remove clothing around burn area
- Immediately cool with flowing water for 5 minutes
- Watch for shivering
- Pat skin dry
- Don't pop blister
- Call doctor
- If this is a large burn, call 911

3rd Degree Burn

Signs and Symptoms
- Charred (Flame)
- White (Hot liquid)

Treatment
LIFE THREAT
- Remove heat source.
- Remove clothing around burn area. Do not attempt to remove fabric sticking to the burn
- Lay infant flat.
- Immediately cool burn site with cool flowing water for 5 minutes.
- Watch for shivering.
- Call 911 immediately

Chemical Burn

Dry Chemical

Brush away chemical with your gloved hand. Wash area with cool, flowing water for 15 minutes. Treat as first, second or third degree burn.

Wet Chemical

Wash away chemical with cool, flowing water for 15 minutes. Treat as first, second or third degree burn.

Bleeding Control

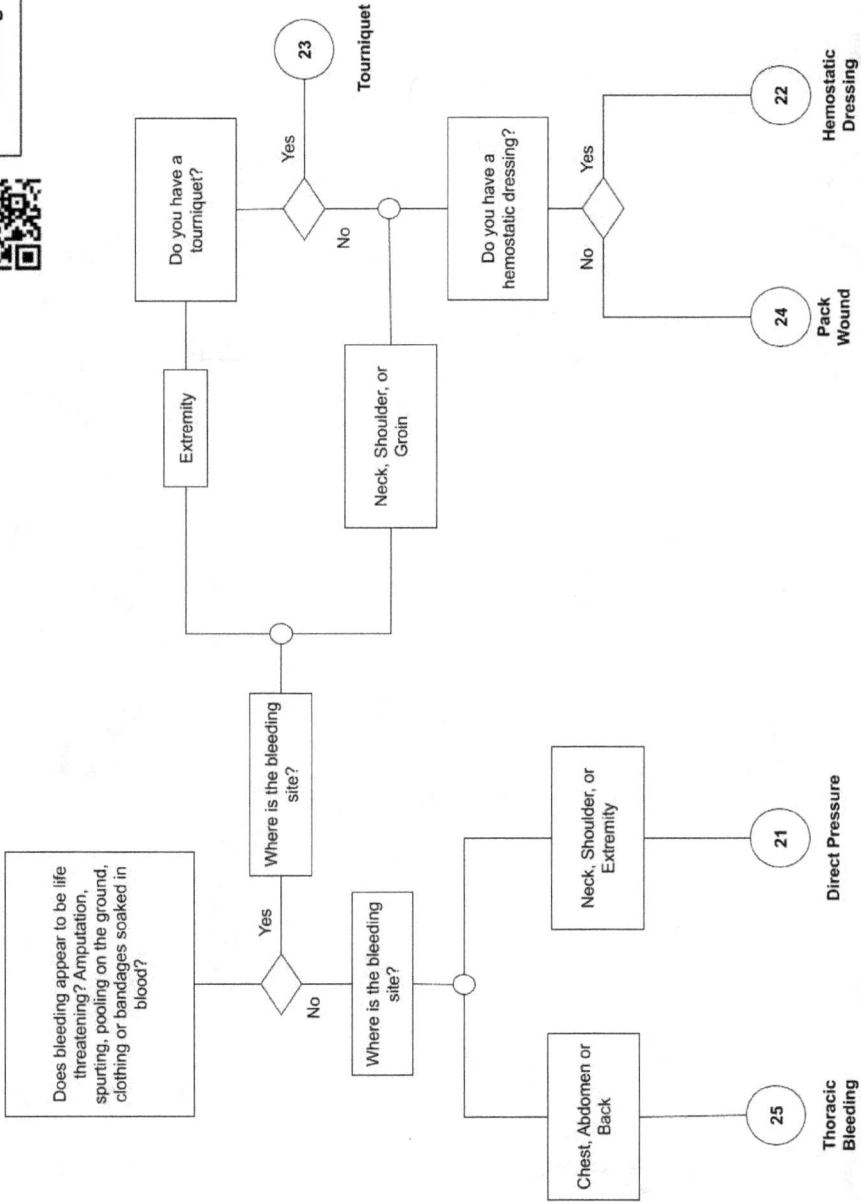

Does bleeding appear to be life threatening? Amputation, spurting, pooling on the ground, clothing or bandages soaked in blood?

Yes → Where is the bleeding site?

- Extremity → Do you have a tourniquet?
  - **Yes** → 23 Tourniquet
  - **No**
- Neck, Shoulder, or Groin → Do you have a hemostatic dressing?
  - **Yes** → 22 Hemostatic Dressing
  - **No** → 24 Pack Wound

No → Where is the bleeding site?

- Neck, Shoulder, or Extremity → 21 Direct Pressure
- Chest, Abdomen or Back → 25 Thoracic Bleeding

Direct Pressure 21

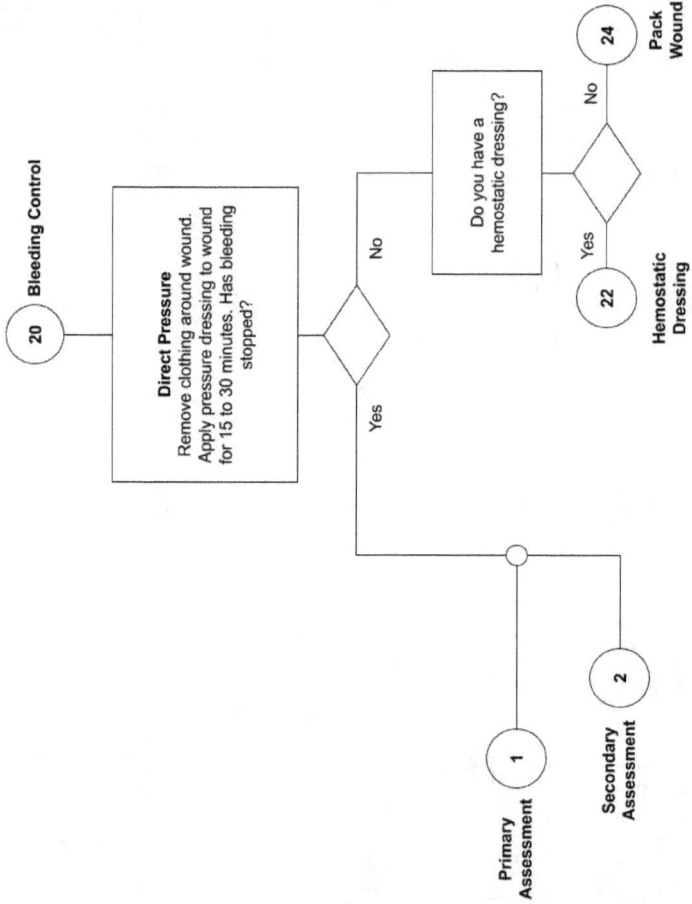

20 **Bleeding Control**

Direct Pressure
Remove clothing around wound. Apply pressure dressing to wound for 15 to 30 minutes. Has bleeding stopped?

Yes

No

Do you have a hemostatic dressing?

Yes

No

22 **Hemostatic Dressing**

24 **Pack Wound**

1 **Primary Assessment**

2 **Secondary Assessment**

Hemostatic Dressing

Alternative
Bleeding Control Methods

- Digital Pressure - Push your gloved finger or thumb into wound, find the bleeding vessel and press it hard against bone.
- Find and and pinch close the bleeding vessel between your gloved forefinger and thumb.

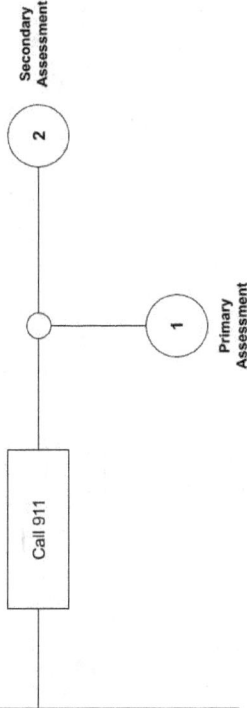

Primary Assessment — 1

Secondary Assessment — 2

Call 911

Bleeding Control — 20

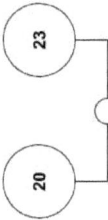

Tourniquet — 23

Hemostatic Dressing

- Remove clothing from bleeding site
- Wipe away any pooled blood
- Pack the wound with a hemostatic dressing.
- Apply steady pressure with both hands directly on top of the bleeding wound.
- Push down as hard as you are able for three minutes
- Hold continuous pressure for 3 minutes
- Reassess to ensure bleeding is controlled.
- Apply second gauze used if initial application fails to stop bleeding
- Leave dressing in place and secure with bandage
- Reassess frequently to monitor for recurrent bleeding
- Call 911

Tourniquet (23)

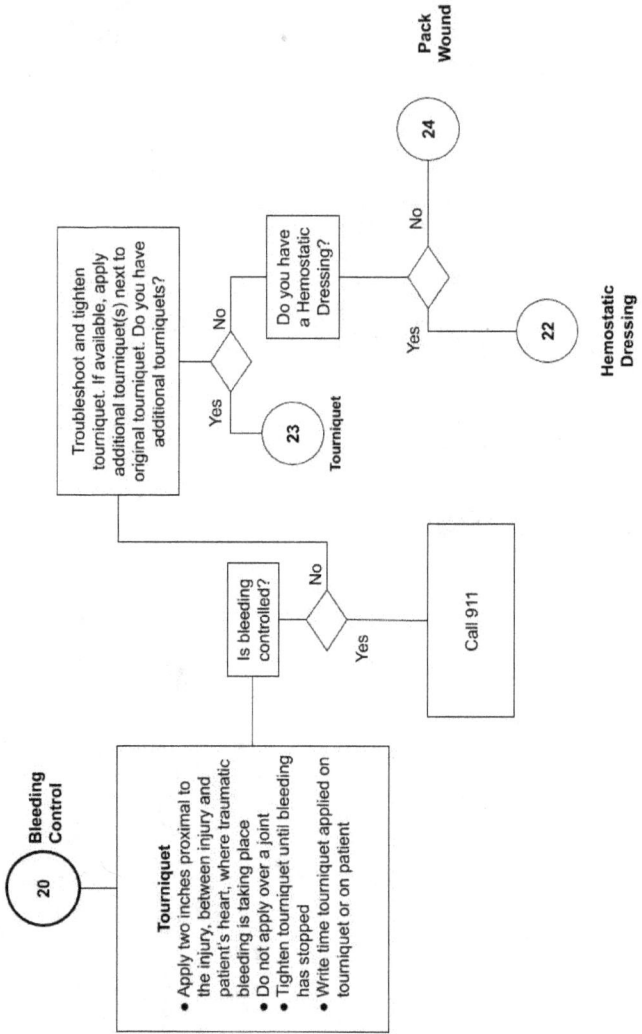

(20) **Bleeding Control**

Tourniquet
- Apply two inches proximal to the injury, between injury and patient's heart, where traumatic bleeding is taking place
- Do not apply over a joint
- Tighten tourniquet until bleeding has stopped
- Write time tourniquet applied on tourniquet or on patient

Is bleeding controlled?

No → **Call 911**

Yes

Troubleshoot and tighten tourniquet. If available, apply additional tourniquet(s) next to original tourniquet. Do you have additional tourniquets?

Yes → (23) **Tourniquet**

No → Do you have a Hemostatic Dressing?

Yes → (22) **Hemostatic Dressing**

No → (24) **Pack Wound**

Pack Wound

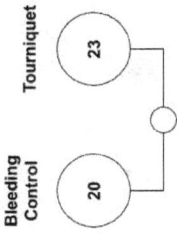

Alternative
Bleeding Control Methods

- Digital Pressure - Push your gloved finger or thumb into wound, find the bleeding vessel and press it hard against bone.
- Find and pinch close the bleeding vessel between your gloved forefinger and thumb.

2 Secondary Assessment

1 Primary Assessment

Call 911

Bleeding Control **Tourniquet**

20   23

Pack Wound

- Remove clothing from bleeding site.
- Wipe away any pooled blood
- Pack the wound with gauze.
- Apply steady pressure with both hands directly on top of the bleeding wound.
- Push down as hard as you are able.
- Hold pressure to stop bleeding.
- Continue pressure until bleeding has stopped or you are relieved by medical responders.

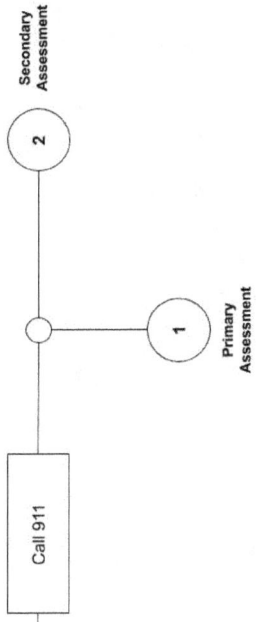

Thoracic Bleeding

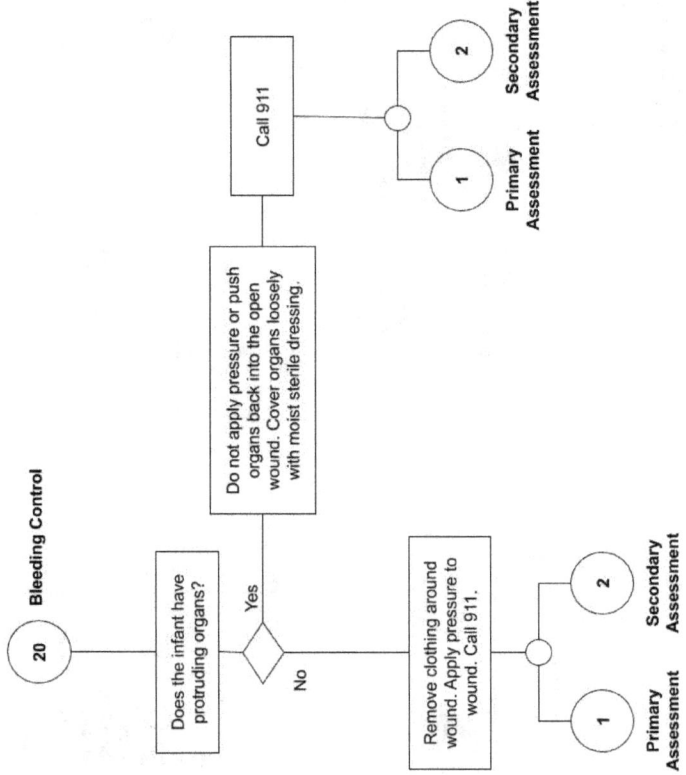

(25)

Bleeding Control

Call 911

(20)

Does the infant have protruding organs?

Yes →

Do not apply pressure or push organs back into the open wound. Cover organs loosely with moist sterile dressing.

No

Remove clothing around wound. Apply pressure to wound. Call 911.

Primary Assessment (1)

Secondary Assessment (2)

Wound Cleaning and Care

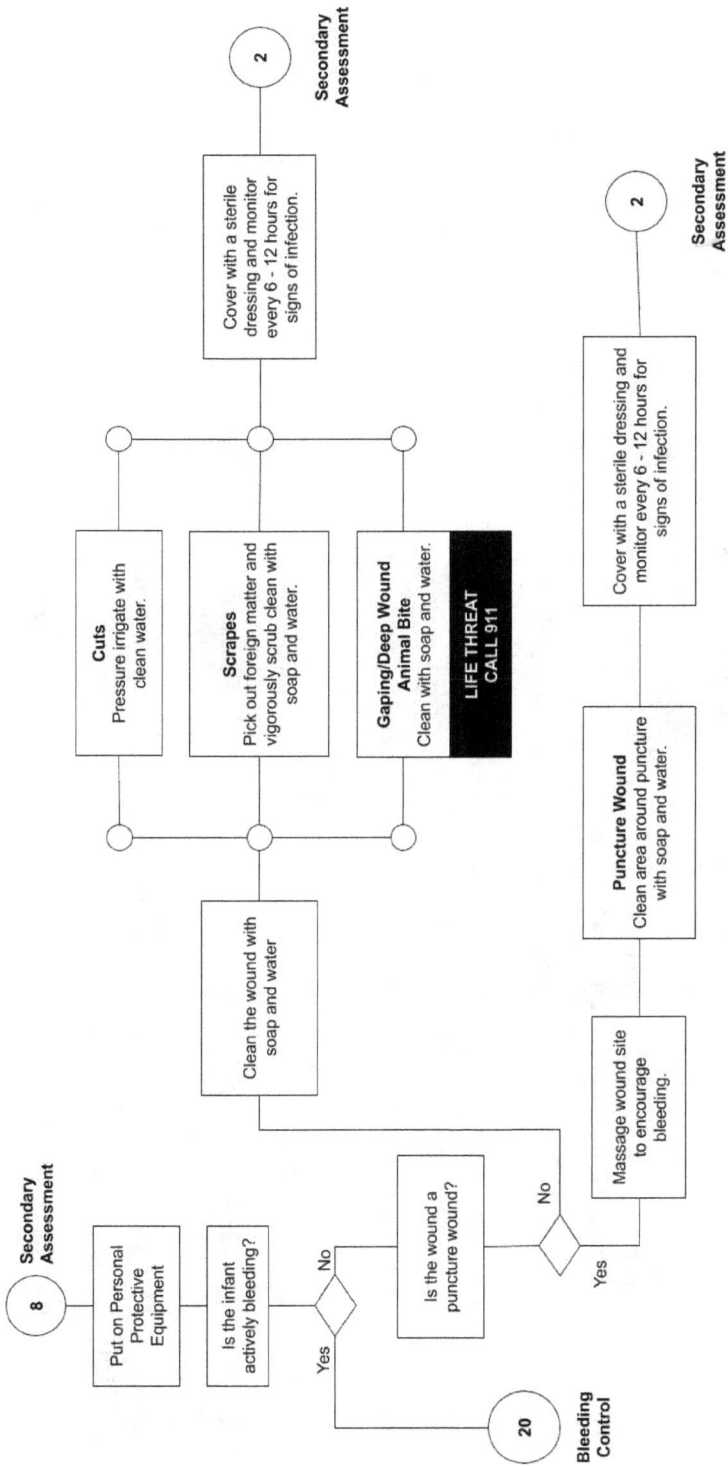

Secondary Assessment
(8)

Put on Personal Protective Equipment

Is the infant actively bleeding?

Yes → (20) **Bleeding Control**

No

Is the wound a puncture wound?

No → Clean the wound with soap and water

Yes → Massage wound site to encourage bleeding.

Clean the wound with soap and water

Cuts
Pressure irrigate with clean water.

Scrapes
Pick out foreign matter and vigorously scrub clean with soap and water.

Gaping/Deep Wound Animal Bite
Clean with soap and water.
LIFE THREAT CALL 911

Cover with a sterile dressing and monitor every 6 - 12 hours for signs of infection.

(2) **Secondary Assessment**

Puncture Wound
Clean area around puncture with soap and water.

Cover with a sterile dressing and monitor every 6 - 12 hours for signs of infection.

(2) **Secondary Assessment**

Sources

"Common Cold in Babies." Mayo Clinic, Mayo Foundation for Medical Education and Research, 21 May 2019, www.mayoclinic.org/diseases-conditions/common-cold-in-babies/symptoms-causes/syc-20351651.

"Cough When to See a Doctor." Mayo Clinic, Mayo Foundation for Medical Education and Research, 21 June 2019, www.mayoclinic.org/symptoms/cough/basics/when-to-see-doctor/sym-20050846.

"Croup: Causes, Symptom, Management & Prevention." Cleveland Clinic, my.clevelandclinic.org/health/diseases/8277-croup.

"Croup." Mayo Clinic, Mayo Foundation for Medical Education and Research, 11 Apr. 2019, www.mayoclinic.org/diseases-conditions/croup/symptoms-causes/syc-20350348.

"Department of Health." Emergency Medical Services and Trauma Systems, www.health.ny.gov/professionals/ems.

"Ear Infection (Middle Ear)." Mayo Clinic, Mayo Foundation for Medical Education and Research, 14 May 2019, www.mayoclinic.org/diseases-conditions/ear-infections/symptoms-causes/syc-20351616.

"Febrile Seizure." Mayo Clinic, Mayo Foundation for Medical Education and Research, 18 June 2019, www.mayoclinic.org/diseases-conditions/febrile-seizure/symptoms-causes/syc-20372522.

"Fever." Mayo Clinic, Mayo Foundation for Medical Education and Research, 21 July 2017, www.mayoclinic.org/diseases-conditions/fever/symptoms-causes/syc-20352759.

"Meningitis." Cleveland Clinic, my.clevelandclinic.org/health/articles/14600-meningitis.

"Meningitis." Mayo Clinic, Mayo Foundation for Medical Education and Research, 8 Jan. 2019, www.mayoclinic.org/diseases-conditions/meningitis/symptoms-causes/syc-20350508.

"Milk Allergy." Mayo Clinic, Mayo Foundation for Medical Education and Research, 6 June 2018, www.mayoclinic.org/diseases-conditions/milk-allergy/symptoms-causes/syc-20375101.

NAEMT. (2016). PHTLS: Prehospital trauma life support (8th ed.). S.l.: JONES & BARTLETT LEARNING.

"Parvovirus Infection." Mayo Clinic, Mayo Foundation for Medical Education and Research, 15 Apr. 2020, www.mayoclinic.org/diseases-conditions/parvovirus-infection/symptoms-causes/syc-20376085.

"Peanut Allergy." Mayo Clinic, Mayo Foundation for Medical Education and Research, 10 Mar. 2020, www.mayoclinic.org/diseases-conditions/peanut-allergy/symptoms-causes/syc-20376175.

"Pediatric Extremity Hemorrhage and Tourniquet Use." JEMS, 24 Sept. 2019, www.jems.com/2018/11/01/pediatric-extremity-hemorrhage-and-tourniquet-use/.

Pollak, A. N., Edgerly, D., McKenna, K., & Vitberg, D. A. (2017). Emergency care and transportation of the sick and injured (11th ed.). Burlington, MA: Jones & Bartlett Learning.

"Respiratory Syncytial Virus (RSV)." Mayo Clinic, Mayo Foundation for Medical Education and Research, 22 July 2017, www.mayoclinic.org/diseases-conditions/respiratory-syncytial-virus/symptoms-causes/syc-20353098.

"Sick Baby? When to Seek Medical Attention." Mayo Clinic, Mayo Foundation for Medical Education and Research, 13 Aug. 2019, www.mayoclinic.org/healthy-lifestyle/infant-and-toddler-health/in-depth/healthy-baby/art-20047793.

"What to Do When Your Newborn Cries." Mayo Clinic, Mayo Foundation for Medical Education and Research, 28 Dec. 2018, www.mayoclinic.org/healthy-lifestyle/infant-and-toddler-health/in-depth/healthy-baby/art-20043859.

"Whooping Cough." Mayo Clinic, Mayo Foundation for Medical Education and Research, 9 Oct. 2019, www.mayoclinic.org/diseases-conditions/whooping-cough/symptoms-causes/syc-20378973.

Alli, Renee A. "Newborne Breathing Noises: Whats Normal & What's Not." WebMD, WebMD, 25 June 2019, www.webmd.com/parenting/baby/your-newborn-babys-breathing-noises#1.

Brennan, Dan. "RSV: Symptoms, Causes, Prevention, Treatments." WebMD, WebMD, 5 Oct. 2019, www.webmd.com/lung/rsv-in-babies#1.

MAJOR TRAUMA GUIDELINES & EDUCATION - VICTORIAN STATE TRAUMA SYSTEM, https://trauma.reach.vic.gov.au/guidelines/paediatric-trauma/secondary-survey

What to Expect. "Treating Burns in Children." What to Expect, What toExpect, 22 Jan. 2019, www.whattoexpect.com/toddler/childhood-injuries/burns-in-children.aspx.

Woollard, M. "5 Assessment and Identification of Paediatric Primary Survey Positive Patients." Emergency Medicine Journal, vol. 21, no. 4, Jan. 2004, pp. 511–517., doi:10.1136/emj.2004.016501.

Index

www.ingramcontent.com/pod-product-compliance
Lightning Source LLC
Chambersburg PA
CBHW070818280326
41934CB00012B/3227